Miracles
with
Minerals

is adapted from the book...

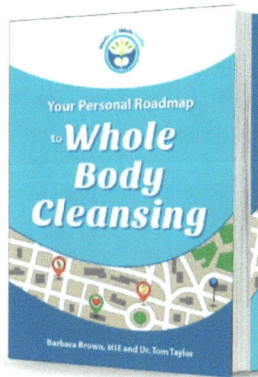

...with additional material written exclusively for
***Miracles* with *Minerals*.**

Your Personal Roadmap to Whole Body Cleansing
is available at www.CleansingRoadmap.com,
where you'll also tap into additional free content!

Miracles with *Minerals*
Feel Better, Look Better, Heal Faster
with the oldest all-natural healing nutrients created by God for the only body you have!

Barbara Brown, MSE and Dr. Tom Taylor

Manufactured in the United States of America

ISBN: 978-1-929921-37-9 (Paperback)
978-1-929921-36-2 (E-Pub)

Published by

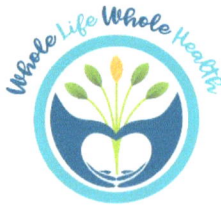

Divine Health is Your Original Design

Trace Minerals PLUS+® is a Registered Trademark of Whole Life Whole Health, LLC.
Lake Dallas, TX 75065 • 940-725-0023

The information contained in this e-book is based on the authors' personal and professional experience and observation and is intended for educational purposes only. It is not intended to diagnose or treat any illness, or to substitute for consulting with a competent health care provider.

"You can trace every sickness, every disease, and every ailment to a mineral deficiency."

Dr. Linus Pauling
Nobel Prize-winning Scientist

We are unspeakably and eternally grateful to the Father of us all, Who created the Earth and everything in it, Who put us here to be nourished in our spirits, souls, and bodies by all that He is and has made for us.

We are also grateful to the thousands of people whom it has been our privilege and honor to serve throughout our journeys. Their trust in us and their commitment to their own health and well-being fueled and sustained our quest for what works 100 percent of the time for everyone.

Science is NOT the source of life and all that feeds it, but science – proper science, that is – agrees with and supports the source of life, and ultimately, everything leads back to the One Who said, when all things were made, "It is good."

God's principles hold true no matter what your gender, race, ethnicity, or beliefs. Your body responds according to its design, not to your desires. When you align yourself with the Father and His design, spiritually, mentally, and physically, illness cannot hold you hostage; healing is inevitable, well-being is unstoppable, and His delight becomes your own.

Sound good?

Let's get on with it, shall we?

Dr. Tom Taylor

TABLE OF CONTENTS

Minerals are essential for all life and without them, life ends. When you are deficient in minerals – and you need more than 70 – you lose quality of life by degrees. The good news is that the opposite is also true: When you replenish your body's supply of minerals daily, you *gain* quality of life in significant ways:

- **Memory improves** – walk into a room and remember why!
- **Immunity increases** – fight off illness easily!
- **Flexibility and mobility improve** – go longer smoother!
- **Sleep improves** – sleep like a baby, even if you're 90!

Help your body run like a well-oiled machine!

Like our friends, family, and clients, we pray that you will also enjoy the benefits above and more!

Blessings and joy on your journey,

Barbara Brown, MSE
Dr. Tom Taylor

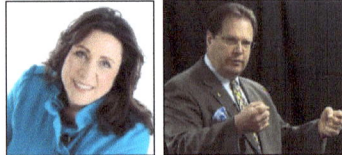

WHAT DO WE TAKE TO STAY YOUNG AND HEALTHY?

This is probably the most frequently asked question we hear.

We do **five things** every day, no matter what, and so do the clients we serve, because we're serious about keeping our bodies humming, with ironclad immune systems and memories like steel traps, sleeping like babies, and otherwise living well in spirit, soul, and body.

Here they are:

The Essential, Non-Negotiable Five

1. TRACE MINERALS PLUS+® Plant-based liquid minerals!

2. JUICE PLUS+® 30 Fruits, Veggies, & grains in capsules!

3. ASEA® Immune-boosting redox signaling supplement!

4. ALKALINE, IONIZED WATER Antioxidizing for *REAL* hydration!

5. BARBARA'S ULTIMATE POWER SHAKE Satisfying & delicious!

You'll find these and every other nutritional product featured in *Your Personal Roadmap to Whole Body Cleansing*, along with specific remedies, everything you'll need for all the cleanses, and other tools too, at our web site:

www.CLEANSINGROADMAP.com

All the products we refer to throughout the book are the same ones we use ourselves. We have tested them extensively, found them to be the best available, and have recommended them to clients for years, with consistently positive results. Our guiding principle for taking or recommending any product is...

> **It doesn't matter what you take.**
> **It matters what your body *does* with what you take.**

The only products we use or recommend are those that withstand the "100% test":

1. The body must be able to *recognize, absorb* and *utilize* the product.

2. It must provide *superior benefit* with little or *no added stress* to the body.

3. It must always test strong on kinesiologic or energetic testing *(aka, "muscle testing")* for anyone, at any age and in any condition. Any product that tests weak is excluded immediately.

Many of the products in these pages may be purchased at "member" prices directly from the companies that market them. We may receive compensation from these companies as a result of your purchase. Any earnings we receive go to support non-profit ministries that help restore broken lives.

WHAT ARE MINERALS AND WHY DO I NEED THEM?

Your body functions according to God's design, not your desire. The natural order works only one way:

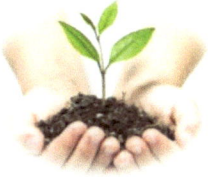

- **The Mineral kingdom feeds the Plant kingdom**
  - **Plants derive minerals from the soil**
- **The Plant kingdom feeds the Animal kingdom**
  - **Animals derive minerals from plant foods**
  - **Animals cannot derive usable minerals directly from the soil**

Minerals are essential nutrients that facilitate more than 10,000 chemical reactions taking place each second at the same time in trillions of cells in your body's tissues, organs...even your bones!

Minerals exist naturally in the soil, but you can't absorb them in this "elemental" or "metallic" form. Humans and animals must derive their minerals from plants, which have broken down material from the soil and rocks into minute, organic particles that are recognizable, absorbable, and usable in your body.

What do minerals do in my body?

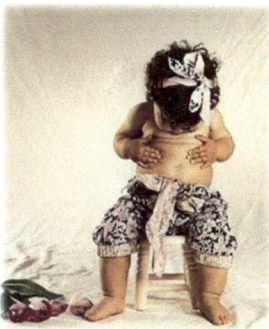

Most of us know that minerals build bones, but minerals are also behind the building up, supporting, cleansing, and tearing down processes that occur every day throughout every organ and tissue. Tens of thousands of enzymes depend on minerals to make chemical reactions occur. Minerals literally make things happen in your body, and without them nothing works.

Dr. Charles Northern, a researcher and MD in the 1930s, said, *"In the absence of minerals, vitamins have no function. Lacking vitamins, the system can make use of the minerals, but lacking minerals, vitamins are useless."*

- ## What is the difference between minerals and "Trace Minerals"?

Minerals are categorized as "major elements," or **Macro Minerals**; "minor elements," and "trace elements" (and recently, "ultra-trace elements") or **Trace Minerals**. Macro minerals are required in relatively large amounts (over 100mg); they include sodium, potassium, magnesium, calcium, phosphorus, and chloride. Minor elements and trace elements are often categorized together as **Trace Minerals**. The name comes from the tiny amounts found in nature and required in the body. Many trace minerals measure more than 1,000 times less than macro minerals, and some are barely measurable at all. Zinc, iron, copper, iodine, and manganese are among the most commonly recognized trace minerals.

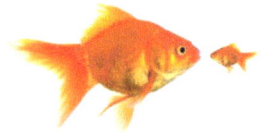

Our soil has been depleted of many minerals since the advent of modern farming in the early 1900s. Even a diet rich in organically grown vegetables and fruit is deficient in minerals that were once plentiful.

- ## What are some signs of a mineral deficiency?

Dr. Linus Pauling, two-time Nobel prize-winning scientist, was quoted as saying, *"You can trace every sickness, every disease, and every ailment to a mineral deficiency."*

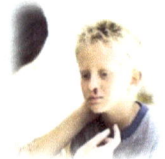

> Some of the landmarks of mineral deficiency include dry skin, acne, poor reflexes, anemia, apathy, general weakness, confusion, sleeplessness, headaches, depression or anxiety, constipation or diarrhea, memory loss, shortness of breath, dandruff, hair loss, susceptibility to illness, poor sense of taste or smell, and hormonal imbalance.

It's easy to see why a mineral supplement has become an important daily requirement for optimal function, disease prevention, and long-term health and well-being.

• Can I get minerals from a daily multivitamin?

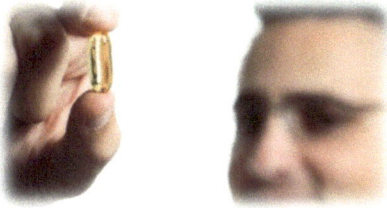

Most vitamin or vitamin/mineral supplements contain only a few of the more than 70 minerals that should be available. Even then, depending on their source and manufacture, only a small amount of any mineral may actually be usable in your body. As one doctor put it, *"Most vitamin/mineral supplements simply become expensive urine."*

• Are there any scientific studies on minerals?

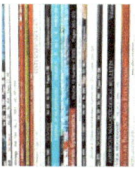

Thousands of scientific studies have been published on the function of specific minerals, their "Recommended Daily Allowance,"* signs of deficiencies and dangers of toxicities, sources, and relative safety.

> ***The RDA has long been recognized as a minimal intake, below which signs of deficiencies are known to occur over time.**

• Why doesn't my doctor recommend or prescribe minerals?

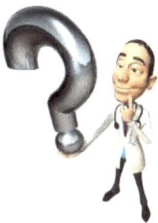

Patients often have more knowledge of nutrition than their doctors. Physicians are trained in pharmacology (drug therapy). Only in that realm are prescriptions permitted legally. Most doctors receive scant training, if any, in the science of nutrition, let alone nutritional supplementation.

Many doctors are aware that "micronutrients," such as vitamins, phytonutrients (nutrients from plants), and minerals, play an important role in human health. Unless your doctor has undertaken extensive study and training in nutrition, he or she is ill-equipped to make dietary or supplement recommendations.

With a few exceptions, medical doctors are not your best sources of knowledge or recommendations regarding nutrition or nutritional supplements.

• What are the differences between mineral supplements?

Mineral supplements come in many forms, from chalk (calcium carbonate) to shells or coral; from rocks to salt or plant deposits; many are extracted – or even worse, synthesized – in laboratories. You'll find tablets, capsules, and various kinds of liquids.

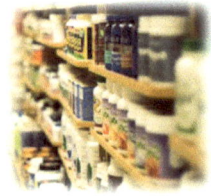

> **The worst part for consumers is that nearly every mineral supplier claims to have the best source, manufacture, purity, absorbability, and efficacy.**

• So, what is the best way to take minerals?

The best mineral "delivery system" we've found is a **liquid**. Tablets, capsules, and even powders, fall short on two counts: First, many contain unnecessary binders or fillers; and second, we find that the **full spectrum** of minerals that ought to be available to your body is present only in liquids.

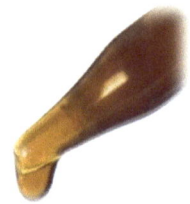

All liquids are not created equal! Beware of products that require ounces per day as a normal amount. You should be able to use up to only a teaspoon per day.

> **Traveling to a country where bacteria or parasites may contaminate the food or water?** You may need to take several teaspoonfuls of liquid minerals per day to avoid dysentery and discourage other parasitic invasions.

• How do I know that minerals are absorbed by my body?

The quickest, simplest, least costly way to know whether you are absorbing the minerals you take is to monitor the signs of mineral deficiency on page 4. Scientists and doctors often dismiss testimonies, or what they call "anecdotal evidence"; costly tests, such as hair analysis, may help "prove" effectiveness; however, our experience is that you know better about how your body feels than any scientist.

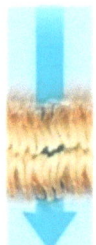

• What effects can I expect from taking minerals?

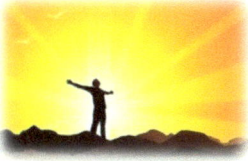

"Expect" is a loaded word, and we can't promise anything from taking liquid minerals. If you're like many we've served over more than two decades, the most obvious signs of improvement include increased energy, improved memory and focus, a higher functioning immune system, and better sleep.

Being deficient in minerals results in a lower quality of life than you deserve, with less resistance to disease, and possibly even a shorter life span. Functioning at the highest level possible in every area of life is impossible to achieve without sufficient minerals. If living at your best and fulfilling the purpose for which you were created is important to you, adding minerals to your daily nutritional regimen is imperative.

• How much of any one mineral should I take?

Drops, NOT ounces!

Most nutrients occur naturally in very small amounts; so, a few drops of the right, full-spectrum, liquid mineral supplement is far better than taking any amount of *one* mineral or group of minerals. The intelligence that God designed in your body will select how much of each nutrient to use at a particular time, so long as you provide *all* the known major, minor and trace elements, in a form your body can *recognize*, *absorb*, and *utilize*.

Studies show that nutrients work best in their natural state, surrounded by other nutrients that work together. For example, we know that calcium, magnesium, phosphorus, and even Vitamin D, are all absorbed and function better when they are all present at the same time, even if the amounts of any one of those minerals is very small.

> The right amount of any one mineral is exactly what your body requires at any given time. The only way to know is to avoid man-made formulas and rely on what God originally created in nature to work together with everything else He created.

WHAT ARE THE BEST SOURCES OF MINERALS?

The best mineral supplements come from ancient plant deposits. Tens of millions of years ago, before anyone farmed anything, the full spectrum of more than 70 minerals was available in the soil. The minerals were taken up by the plants that grew abundantly at the time; as those plants died and decomposed, they naturally replenished the soil with the same minerals. The cycle was repeated over millions of years until an enormous amount of naturally organic material was built up, called "humic shale" or "humic clay," containing an important substance, called "fulvic acid."

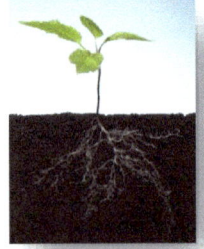

Two Amazing Facts

Minerals from soil, rocks, salts, or shells – anything other than plants – are useless and even toxic to your body, because they are in an "elemental" or "metallic" state.

Plants miraculously change unusable, or otherwise toxic, minerals into a form your body can recognize, absorb, and utilize exactly as God intended.

- **How do minerals become liquid?**

Today, we can tap an ancient, composted plant deposit – which looks like coal – dry it until it becomes a sandy consistency, drip water through it – s l o w l y – and produce a liquid, called a "colloid." This amber-colored liquid appears to be a clear solution, but it contains millions of mineral particles so small that they are always suspended in the water. This liquid also contains "fulvic acid," which is created by microbial action between the soil and the roots where plants absorb these vital nutrients. Fulvic acid gives liquid minerals a kind of "living" property.

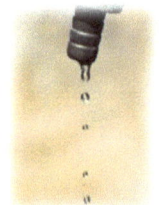

• **Do liquid minerals contain all the nutrients I need?**

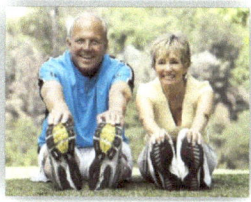

The subject of how many nutrients are required by human beings is controversial and hotly debated in scientific circles even in the 21st century. Amazingly, as late as the mid 1980's, scientists added nutrients such as chromium, nickel, tin, vanadium, and boron, to a list of only 15 minerals considered as essential or beneficial. The exact benefits of at least 55 other minerals are still unknown or unstudied.

> **Before anyone farmed anything, more than 70 minerals were present to support human life!**

Liquid minerals, from the right source, can provide all the minerals that are needed in small amounts; other food sources are required for minerals that you need in much greater amounts.

> **Liquid minerals do *NOT* supply *ALL* the nutrients you need – they supply nutrients you absolutely *MUST* have and *WON'T* find anywhere else!**

• **What mineral supplement do WE use every day?**

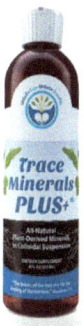

We use **TRACE MINERALS PLUS+®**, which comes from people we know and trust, whose family pioneered much of the earliest work on minerals for both agricultural use and human consumption. They have kept pure the prehistoric plant deposit source they own. We have a long history together and are grateful to label their product for our professional and private clients. Our *"Essential, Non-Negotiable Five"* for daily health is on Page 1.

> **Each day, we make *"Barbara's Ultimate Power Breakfast"* that contains between 20-40 drops of minerals. Once a week, we substitute a ROYAL FLUSH®, which you can learn more about in *Your Personal Roadmap to Whole Body Cleansing*, and at www.CleansingRoadmap.com.**

10

WHAT TO WATCH OUT FOR WITH LIQUID MINERALS

• **How long do liquid minerals last?**

This is one of our favorite questions. Think of it this way: If your liquid mineral supplement is already 60-70 million years old, how much older can it possibly get in *your* lifetime? This is *NOT* true, however, for mineral supplements, such as tablets, capsules, powders, and many other liquids, which carry expiration dates.

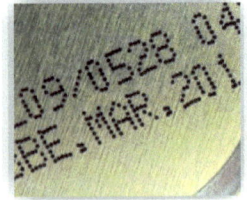

> **If your mineral supplement has an expiration date on it, consider a different supplement!**

• **Are liquid minerals organic?**

Plant-derived minerals are naturally organic, not to be confused with "certified organic." The plant deposit that produces TRACE MINERALS PLUS+® existed long before humans farmed anything, let alone before the use of toxic chemicals associated with modern commercial farming. As much as certified organic farming helps reclaim and maintain the purity of the soil's microbiological activity, the full spectrum of minerals, which was lacking when the organic farmer began tilling the soil, is still lacking.

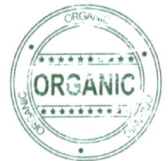

> **Farmers and home gardeners can replenish their soil's mineral-rich environment by mixing TRACE MINERALS PLUS+® directly into their soil!**

The original discoverer of TRACE MINERALS PLUS+® once supplied minerals to farmers who found that their crops grew better, resisted disease and pests without resorting to toxic chemicals, and contained nutrients not found with other "fertilizers"!

● **Are liquid minerals safe for all ages?**

We can confidently testify to the safety of TRACE MINERALS PLUS+® after well over two decades of experience in using liquid minerals and recommending them to clients with 100 percent positive results, no matter what their age or condition. TRACE MINERALS PLUS+®, together with other responsible habits (discussed in *Your Personal Roadmap to Whole Body Cleansing*), helps establish and maintain an iron-clad immune system. We've discovered that no "unfriendly" organism can survive in the presence of these minerals, but they never hurt, and only support, the "friendly" organisms you need to thrive.

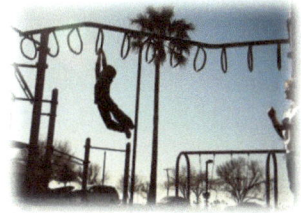

● **Why would liquid minerals contain lead, arsenic, and mercury?**

Everyone knows that aluminum is toxic to humans, right? Yet, from 1970 and 1984, aluminum, bromine, vanadium, and nickel – even arsenic and lead – were found in human milk, together with at least 56 other trace minerals, suggesting that human beings *need* minerals that were once considered toxic or of little to no benefit.

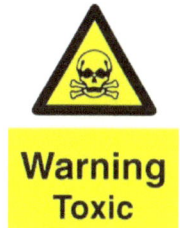

Elements like those above, and others, may be toxic in their elemental or metallic state, but when plants "digest" minerals, their electrochemical structure changes into forms that are not only nontoxic to animals and humans, but are essential to carry on activities within your body that we still don't fully understand.

God designed the natural balance between and among all the elements. We prefer to rely on His wisdom rather than that of any human, no matter how educated.

We will not endorse or recommend, much less use, supplements which a company has altered to suit its idea of what is "safe." The consequences of disturbing naturally balanced elements have often proven far worse than any supposed benefit.

OTHER IMPORTANT POINTS ABOUT LIQUID MINERALS

● **Liquid minerals stain!**

If the liquid gets on fabric, use a spot remover, and wash it immediately. With some fabrics, this may not even work. It's best to keep everything away from liquid minerals except what you want them on!

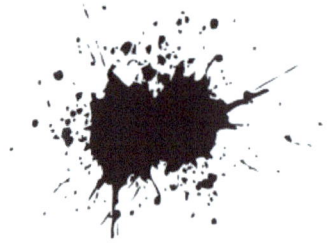

● **Never heat liquid minerals!**

Heat kills the vital properties of liquid minerals; however, a few drops in bath water can help neutralize the chlorine in tap water.

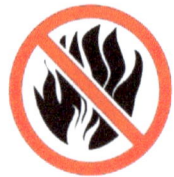

● **Liquid minerals are highly astringent.**

Never use liquid minerals directly in the eyes! If your eyes are exposed, flush with water immediately.

● **Liquid minerals are super bitter!**

We've never chewed on a rusty fence, but that's the image that comes to mind. You can gain first-hand experience with the bitter taste of liquid minerals by putting a drop on your tongue. YUCK!

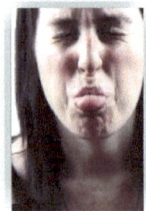

● **Liquid minerals can sting.**

When applying liquid minerals to open wounds, especially for kids and animals, mix 1 drop of minerals with 3-4 drops of water.

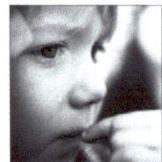

● **No "bad guy bugs" can live with liquid minerals.**

Liquid minerals naturally kill and repel unfriendly bacteria and viruses, but they'll never hurt you when used properly.

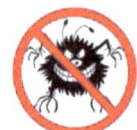

HOW TO GET THE MOST FROM TRACE MINERALS PLUS+®

Health and wellness are the natural consequences of taking charge and taking care of your body, mind, and spirit. Physically, your goal ought to be to cultivate an internal environment that promotes and supports your total well-being, and vigorously defends against environmental invaders.

> **Just 20 drops a day of TRACE MINERALS PLUS+® can help you achieve that goal.**

Mix **20 drops** (1/4 teaspoon) into shakes, smoothies, or eight ounces of fresh fruit juice once a day (we find that orange and grapefruit work best). You'll be replenishing what *should* be in the food you eat but isn't, and what your body desperately needs.

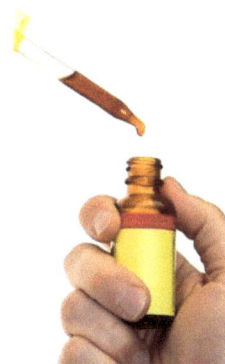

TRACE MINERALS PLUS+® is an accurate name, unlike other products, because the plant deposit from which these liquid minerals are derived contains a **complete spectrum** of all-natural trace and ultra-trace elements,

> *"20 drops a day keeps the doctor away!"*

plus minor and macro minerals. In addition, the fulvic acid* in TRACE MINERALS PLUS+® gives this solution some truly astonishing properties:

- **Energizes water and makes it better able to carry nutrients into, and carry waste products away from, your cells.**

- **Alerts and strengthens the immune system**

- **Helps neutralize toxins**

- **Neutralizes viruses**

- **Highly absorbable and bio-active**

- **Acts as a natural antibiotic, antimicrobial and antiviral agent**

*see page 8

FIRST AID WITH TRACE MINERALS PLUS+®

TRACE MINERALS PLUS+® has tremendous healing properties that we have been privileged to experience firsthand, and witness in the lives of countless individuals and families over more than two decades.

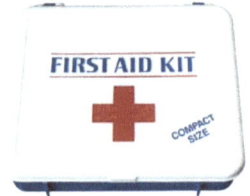

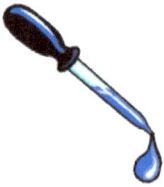

The following are some of the most common applications for which TRACE MINERALS PLUS+® have proven to deliver effective first aid.

- **Cuts**

After cleaning a wound, put a drop of TRACE MINERALS PLUS+® (or more, depending on wound size) directly on the cut or wound. This will most often cauterize the bleeding. Deeper wounds may require bandaging and pressure, but TRACE MINERALS PLUS+® will help cauterize and clean the wound until medical attention can be obtained.

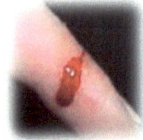

- **Burns**

Put TRACE MINERALS PLUS+® on any burn area, followed by ice. Do this twice. After the second application of minerals and ice, no blister will raise and often you won't even be able to find the burn!

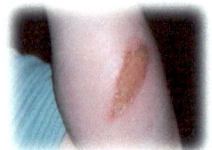

- **Sore Throats**

Put 4-5 drops of TRACE MINERALS PLUS+® in 1-2 oz. of water, gargle and swallow. Once may be enough if you catch it early. If not, repeat 3-6 times per day. The condition should clear up in 1-2 days (even Thrush and Strep Throat).

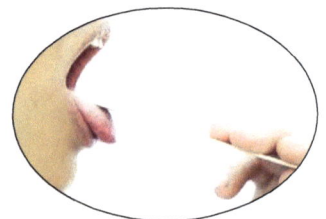

• Sinus Infections

Put 4-6 drops of **TRACE MINERALS PLUS+**® in an ounce of saline solution (salt water), with a cap that allows you to create a nasal spray. Spray and inhale the mixture through each nostril into the sinuses. Get tissues ready because the sludge that you'll blow out is unbelievable! For impacted sinuses, more than one application may be needed, but they'll often clear within 24 hours. This method works for sinus congestion too!

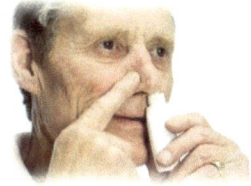

• Boils and Skin Eruptions

Use just like cuts and wounds. Wet a bandage pad with 2-3 drops of **TRACE MINERALS PLUS+**® and cover the area. Do this twice a day for as long as needed. Boils usually clear up in a few days.

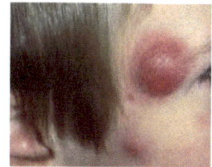

• Tooth Abscesses (or impacted teeth)

Soak a Q-Tip® with 3-4 drops of **TRACE MINERALS PLUS+**® and rub into the gum line at the involved tooth *(Note: You will taste the minerals)*. Repeat this a few times a day until you can get to your dentist, or until the abscess clears or resolves itself; but don't wait more than a couple of days.

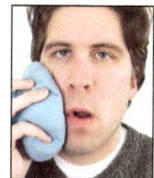

■ **Additional Help:** After applying **TRACE MINERALS PLUS+**®, open a capsule of probiotics and massage into the gum line.

• Cold and Chancre Sores

Apply 1 drop of **TRACE MINERALS PLUS+**® directly to the area. Use a Q-Tip® if you like. Liquid minerals will stain external sores, but they can clear up in less than 24 hours. For internal sores, use as described for tooth remedies above and repeat as needed.

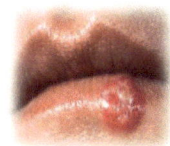

• Internal Bleeding

Mix 1 teaspoon of TRACE MINERALS PLUS+® in orange or grapefruit juice, and drink daily for 3 days. If the stool turns black, continue for 21 days. Stool should change to brown within that time. If not, seek medical help.

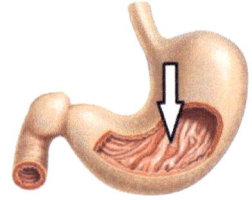

• Sunburn

Apply TRACE MINERALS PLUS+® directly to the sunburned area (use a soaked cotton pad). If the area is quite large, put 1 tablespoon of TRACE MINERALS PLUS+® in a tub of water that is just warm enough to get in, and bathe for 10-20 minutes. You may need to repeat this daily until the burn heals, depending on its severity.

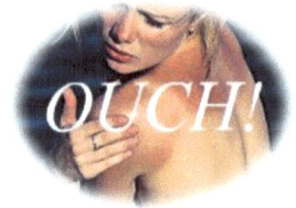

• Hemorrhoids

If hemorrhoids aren't bleeding, put 3-4 drops of TRACE MINERALS PLUS+® on a single square of toilet paper folded in quarters. Apply the minerals directly on the hemorrhoids with pressure; then apply ointment over the area (our favorite is "Neem" ointment). For bleeding hemorrhoids, make a "sitz bath" of warm water and a teaspoon of TRACE MINERALS PLUS+®. Sit in the solution for at least 5 minutes and repeat twice daily until tissues heal enough to use the procedure above, (usually 1-2 days).

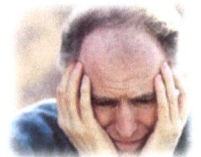

• Systemic Yeast Infections (Candida)

Use ¼ teaspoon of TRACE MINERALS PLUS+® three times a day in water (remember, this tastes bitter). Avoid *ALL* dairy, grains, refined sugar, and fruit. This can take several weeks to clear up.

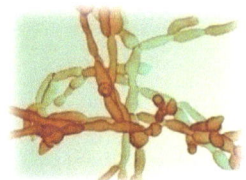

- **Vaginal Yeast and Vaginitis**

Prepare a douche container filled with sterile saline. Add 4 drops of TRACE MINERALS PLUS+® and apply 1-2 times per day. This will often clear up even the most raging infections in 1-3 days.

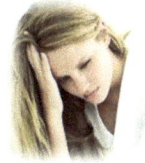

- **Ear Infections**

Put 1-2 drops of TRACE MINERALS PLUS+® directly into the affected ear, pack gently with cotton, and apply moist heat (hot water bottles work well), while lying on the affected side. Repeat 2-3 times a day. Infections often clear in a day or less.

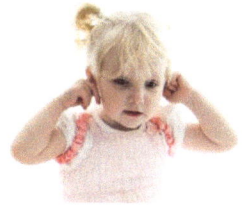

- **Traveling**

Take *at least* a teaspoon of TRACE MINERALS PLUS+® per day when traveling to avoid diarrhea from unfamiliar water and foods.

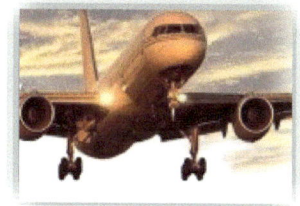

Share your MINERAL MIRACLES with us!

What uses can *you* find for TRACE MINERALS PLUS+® that work 100% of the time?

Email them to Stories@MiracleswithMinerals.com

We'll say, *"Thank You"* by sending
Your Personal Roadmap to Whole Body Cleansing
as a PDF download!

THE ORIGIN AND HISTORY OF TRACE MINERALS PLUS+®

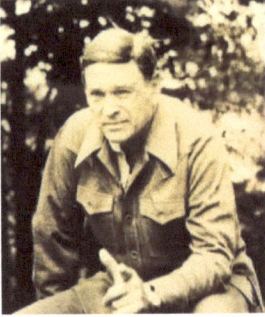

John Scott needed help to make the sandy soil of his Florida land more fertile for his citrus groves, his blueberry bushes, and his ornamental fern crops. It seemed obvious to him that anything grown on healthy, rich soil would be more disease resistant, have increased nutritional value, and have a longer shelf life after it was harvested. Fortunately for us today, Mr. Scott also wanted to find a solution that would free him from any dependence on chemical fertilizers and pesticides.

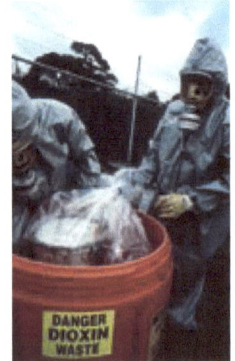

During World War II, Mr. Scott worked at a chemical defense plant in Houston, Texas, where many petroleum-based products were being developed. The scientists at the plant constantly warned the men who worked there not to let a drop of the substances they were handling touch them, because of their high toxicity levels. One of the substances that Mr. Scott heard the scientists name was dioxin. When he learned that one of the pest control measures farmers were using on food crops included the random spraying of dioxin and other toxic substances, such as DDT, he became understandably alarmed.

After World War II, Mr. Scott began researching natural solutions to nourish the soil of his own farmland in Florida. He learned of a group of men who owned a unique mineral deposit that had been discovered in 1948 in the Southeastern United States. The men were using the mineral deposit, often called "humic clay" or "humic shale," in compost as a soil supplement.

Humic clay deposits formed in the virgin soil of the late Cretaceous and early Tertiary periods, 60-70 million years ago. As pre-historic vegetation absorbed the inorganic minerals in the ground and converted them into naturally organic minerals, the plants enjoyed robust growth in lush forests. These nutrient-rich plants lived and died in cycles that repeated over a period of millions of years, composting layer upon layer to form what we know today as, "humic clay" or "humic shale." Perhaps the richest source of minerals that your body can recognize, absorb, and utilize today is found in these ancient, nutrient-rich deposits.

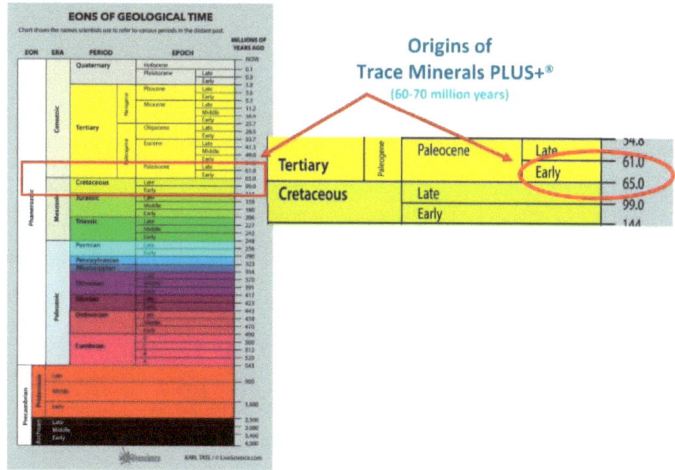

The process of prehistoric plants taking up inorganic minerals from the soil and converting them into organic minerals involved or produced a substance called, "fulvic acid."* The high fulvic acid content of prehistoric soil is one of the properties that makes liquid minerals bioavailable to plants and, through them, to animals. Fulvic acid acts as an electrolyte, providing a constant trickle of electricity to living cells. Fulvic acid contains living properties that seem to account for the often astonishing healing properties of plant-based, liquid minerals derived from humic clay.

How Fulvic Acid is Formed

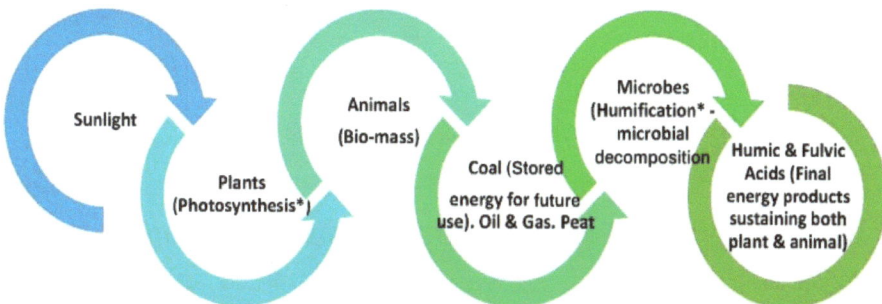

*You can read more about fulvic acid and access an extensive list of scientific references at www.supremefulvic.com/resources.php.

CAUTION: We do *not* recommend fulvic acid as an isolated supplement, such as on the web site above. Any naturally occurring substance is changed when it is isolated from the constituents that surround it in nature (i.e., the soil or plants in which it is normally found and the minerals with which it normally interacts). This is why isolated nutrients, such as Vitamin E or beta-carotene, for example, never work as well as when they are left intact in a carrot. Studies have demonstrated that these isolated nutrients can even have detrimental effects on human health.

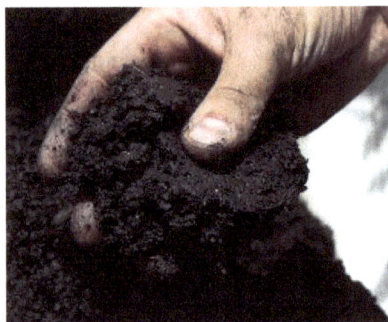

The "vein" of humic clay that John Scott investigated was found in an area of the Deep South, from about 12 inches below the topsoil to about 8-10 feet or more below the surface. Once a small portion of the humic clay was extracted, it required a year to "cure" simply by being left outside to dry. Once this curing process was complete, the once coal-like, hard mineral substance became like fine sand in texture. Oddly, one person who tasted the cured mineral powder expected it to be gritty in his mouth; instead, he said it dissolved as quickly as cotton candy.

Horse trainers administered the cured mineral "powder" to their racehorses as part of their feed, and applied it to injuries and wounds, all with excellent results. In fact, some breeders discovered that their "trace mineral horses" had bone densities three times that of other horses after only six months. Farmers found that the fertility rates of their cattle increased from 78% to an astonishing 98%

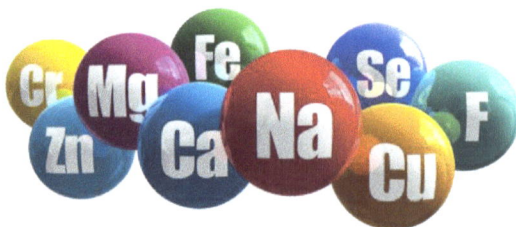

when their feed included some of the cured mineral product. A local university found that shrimp raised in an environment that included a little of the mineral powder grew much larger than those raised in tanks without the minerals. People were also experiencing benefits from using the mineral clay in even tiny amounts as a nutritional supplement and as a topical remedy. In Hungary, where another humic clay deposit is found, one study of 1100 children with eczema given only the fulvic acid component in humic trace minerals showed that all were clear of the skin disorder in nine months.

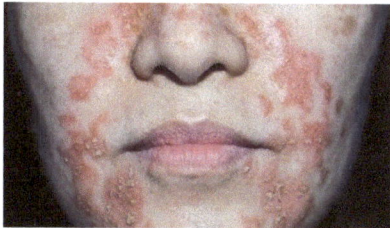

John Scott bought the mineral deposit from the group of owners in 1975 and started Scott's Nutritional Services. Rice and soybean farmers were eager to spread the mineral powder over their fields, but the FDA abruptly banned all interstate transport across state lines. Not long after, a poultry farmer who agreed to test the minerals on his chickens in powder and liquid form had a fire break out mysteriously in the office where he kept the test results. Although the fire-proof cabinet saved the test documents and a second trial was performed, another fire broke out. Suspiciously, the cabinet was found open, and all records were destroyed. The poultry farmer finally decided not to pursue a non-chemical, alternative way to raise his chickens.

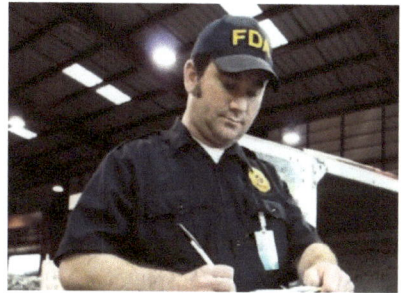

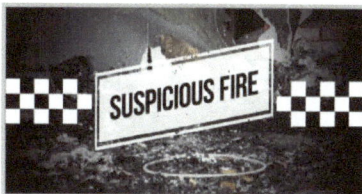

These setbacks did not stop Mr. Scott from continuing to research and teach others about the importance of proper mineral balance in the soil, in livestock, and in human nutrition, until his death in 1986.

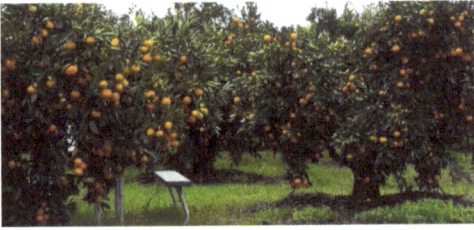

As a result of his earliest applications of humic clay in its powdered form to his Florida soil, Mr. Scott observed significant increases in his crop yields and that his plants were astonishingly resistant to disease and pests. He also found that the nutrient density of his blueberry and citrus fruits was evident in their increased sweetness and longer shelf life once they were harvested. Even his ornamental ferns were larger and hardier than those grown before he introduced the minerals to the soil.

Among John Scott's discoveries was that trace minerals in liquid form was easier to control in agricultural use and demonstrated tremendous benefits in human and animal nutrition. The naturally "bacteriostatic" property of trace minerals stopped the growth of bacteria that could easily contaminate food and water supplies. This important insight echoed the experience of early American pioneers, who learned to place silver coins in canteens to purify their drinking water.

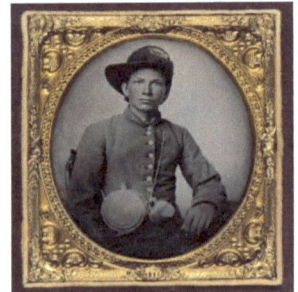

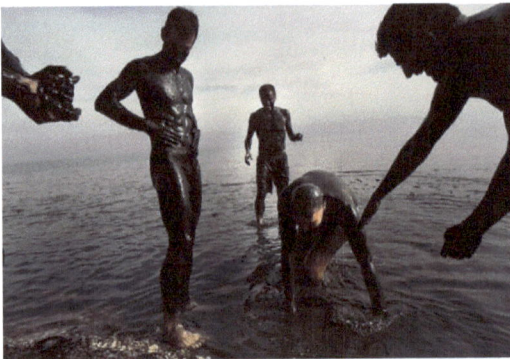

Minerals in humic clay have been used for centuries by native people who would heal wounds by packing them with clay from riverbanks. To this day, people flock to mineral hot springs and pay thousands of dollars to immerse themselves in mud baths for their soothing and even curative properties.

TRACE MINERALS PLUS+® is processed today using John Scott's original specifications and standards.

An age-old dripping process, using only cool, filtered spring water, turns the dried, powered clay into a highly concentrated mineral-rich liquid. This slow-dripping process "activates" the fulvic acid and disperses 74 minerals into a "colloidal suspension" containing minute particles that can't be seen with the naked eye and that don't settle out of their water carrier.

As long as TRACE MINERALS PLUS+® is not exposed to excessive heat, its properties virtually never expire. Any residue found in the bottom of a bottle is undissolved humic clay and any yellow-brownish crust at the spout is dried sulfur; both are perfectly harmless.

HOW TRACE MINERALS HELPED SAVE MY LIFE

If you ever experience a ruptured appendix – and I pray you never do! – you'll need serious help to recover from the literal dumping of toxic waste into your abdominal cavity. It's an experience I had in 1998 and I almost didn't survive. When they saw the extent of the internal contamination created by the rupture, the team of doctors who performed emergency surgery did not expect me to live through it, much less recover my health.

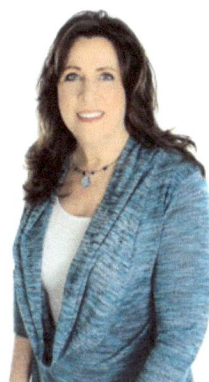

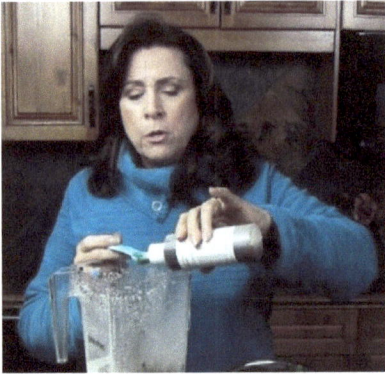

The experience compelled me not only to take charge of my health, but also to discover the means necessary to make my body too healthy for any illness or disease process to gain a foothold. My search led me, among many other destinations, to a health food store in Dallas, Texas, where a holistic practitioner steered me to a plastic bottle of liquid minerals containing more than 70 elements, many of which I had never heard of before and about which I knew nothing.

I began taking a few drops a day of the liquid minerals in juice, and I gradually increased the amount to as much as a full teaspoon a day while performing a nutritional cleansing program called the Royal Flush®. John Scott had developed this unique detoxifying intestinal cleansing system with the help of the Dallas health food store's owner.

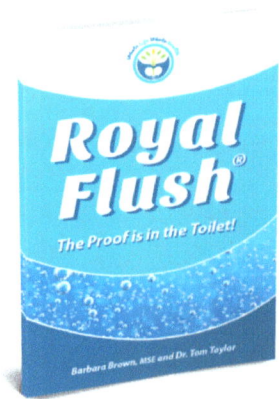

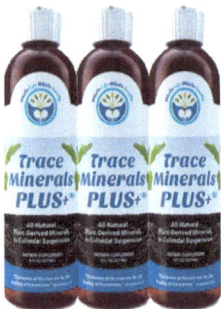

Along my journey, I met John Scott's daughter, who continued her father's work and who graciously shared the information for this report. When Whole Life Whole Health, LLC. was formed in 2008, the first product we offered our clients was Scott's Trace Minerals. This became trademarked in 2014 as TRACE MINERALS PLUS+®.

Learn more at TraceMineralsPLUS.com.

TONS MORE "HOW TO'S" AND OTHER TREASURES
When you visit *www.CleansingRoadmap.com*

➤ **VIDEOS** – Access 20 videos answering the most important questions about Nutritional Cleansing and bonus videos which ensure your success. We've done the work. Just watch and follow along!

➤ **ACTION GUIDES** – Let us walk you through the steps that lead to success, whether it's losing weight, getting through caffeine withdrawal, or getting the most from your cleanses!

➤ **RESOURCES AND BEST SOURCES** – Find out what's worth watching and who's worth tracking! If you want to take your precious time searching through mountains of information and countless web sites, trying to find the stuff you need and the information you seek, be our guest, but chances are, we've already found most of what you'll need.

➤ **RECOMMENDED READING** – When it comes to health and wellness, authorities abound and very few agree. The good news is that the list is fairly short, and the authors we trust get results. Have an authority you'd like us to check out? Let us know. We'll tell you what we think!

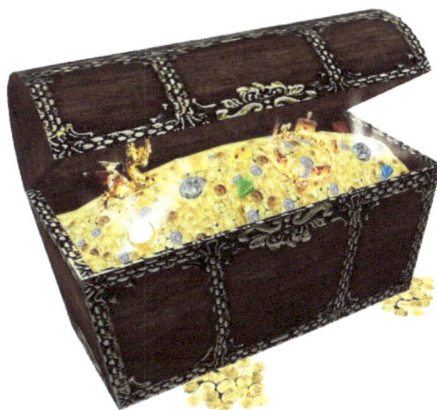

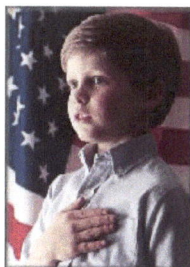

HERE'S OUR PLEDGE: We will *ONLY* share what passes the "100% test" we defined on Page 2. When anything is found to create more stress than benefit, we won't waste your time.

"…let your word be 'Yes, Yes,' or 'No, No.'" (Matthew 5:37)

1. You'll get instant access to **Your Personal Roadmap to Whole Body Cleansing** as a full color PDF download.

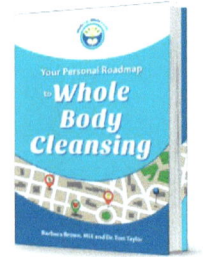

2. Plus, a simple Food Combining Guide.

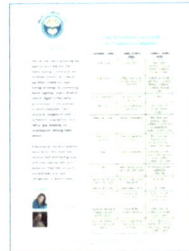

3. "Where to Find it" – 25 point-and-click sources for all the products you'll find in the book.

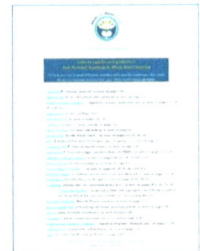

4. Follow-up links to all the free additional content promised in the book!

You'll receive your *FREE* bonuses automatically through your exclusive online environment for True Health-Seekers!!

Order Trace Minerals PLUS+®
at www.TraceMineralsPLUS.com

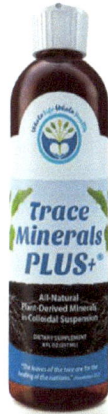

"...your body is a temple of the Holy Spirit in you, which you have from God, and you are not your own. For you are bought with a price. By all means glorify God in your body." (1 Corinthians 6:19-20)

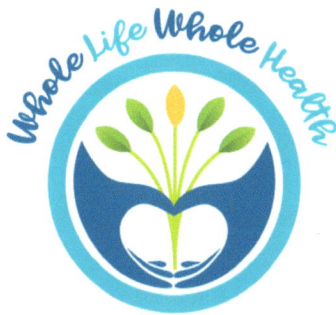

Divine Health is Your Original Design

www.WholeLifeWholeHealth.com

www.ingramcontent.com/pod-product-compliance
Lightning Source LLC
Chambersburg PA
CBHW060854270326
41934CB00002B/128